Practical Workout, Nutrition, and Supplement Guide

Comprehensive 9 Months Holistic Lifestyle Protocol

Resti Tito H. Villarino, R.N.

Dedication

Mau

Niño

Sugar

Angel

TGBTG

Table of Contents

I. The Body As a Tool

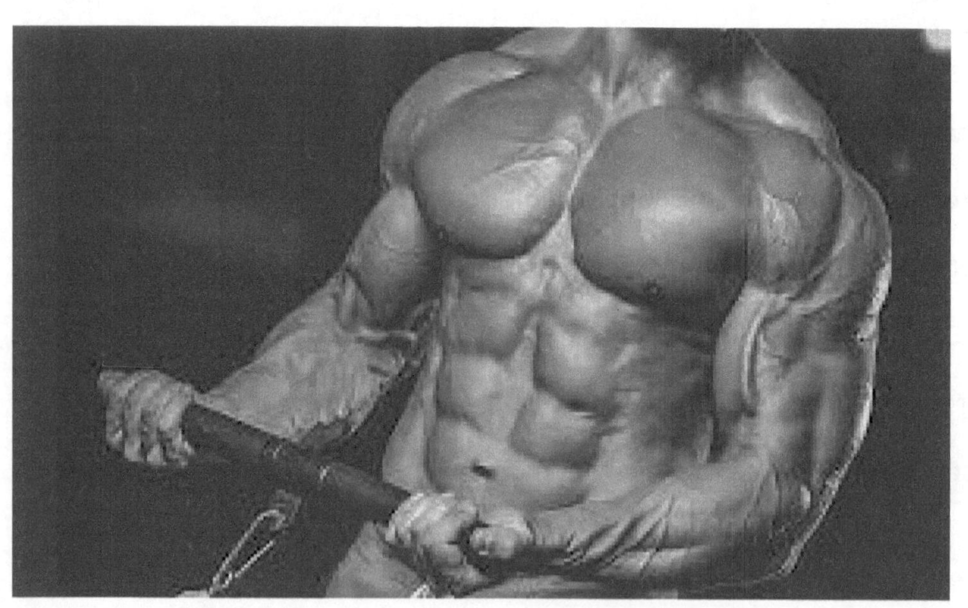

Chapter I. Body as a Tool

Importance of Working-out towards Holistic Health

One of the most challenging task of Introducing a holistic lifestyle regimen is what, who, where, when, how, and why to start. We dig thru literature and the internet to provide us with a complete and comprehensive knowledge and skill set in order for us to be guided accordingly. But due to inconveniences and confusing too-much-information, we ended up not knowing what to do. Thus, with this compendium of routines, nutrition, and supplement guide, the author aims to bring out the best version of YOU.

Major Body Parts involve in Working-out

There are six major body parts in a holistic workout regimen. The Chest and Triceps, Back and Biceps, Shoulder and Legs. It is important to include all these functional body parts to achieve a balance body proportion. Aside from symmetrical body proportions, another advantage of doing exercises involving all these body parts is that it helps increase cardiovascular endurance which facilitates in fat metabolism resulting in a low-body fat percentage.

All exercises should be done six times a week. The seventh day is intended for rest and recovery. It is important to monitor the weight (approximately 5 to 10 pounds increase per week so as to avoid muscle plateau). You have to chart your progress on the DEVELOPMENT CHART provided here. Starting weight is 5 lbs. (recommended) or you may start at 10 lbs. depending on your preference but make sure to consult your doctor before doing any of these exercises to avoid unwanted health effects. Recording is done daily and should perform each exercise PROPERLY and in a SLOW yet INTENSIVE and FOCUSED manner. Duration of the exercise is usually 2 hrs. maximum but if you can complete this exercises within an hour the better because it helps maximize muscle recovery. PHASE I Exercises are done for the First Month. PHASE II is done the following month for the NEXT three Months. PHASE III is done after three months until the sixth month. PHASE IV is done sixth month towards the ninth month. Then back to PHASE I.A again but this time with weight increments from the previous PHASE I. It is a CYCLING METHOD approach because the end goal is to confuse the muscles to provide with maximum effect in a 9 month period. This approach is no shortcut at all but with whole-hearted efforts you will REAP the RESULTS.

PHASE I.
Date:
Duration: 2 hours or less
Current weight in Kg.:
End- Goal: *Lean Body Mass*
A. Warm –Up (Light Stretching) 3 minutes

B. Squat (6 sets= 13 reps, 13, 11, 11, 11, 15)
1st week weight:
2nd week weight:
3rd week weight:
4th week weight:

C. Military Press (6 sets= 13 reps, 13, 11, 11, 11, 15)
1st week weight:
2nd week weight:
3rd week weight:
4th week weight:

D. Flat Bench Press (6 sets= 13 reps, 13, 11, 11, 11, 15)
1st week weight:
2nd week weight:
3rd week weight:
4th week weight:

E. Close Grip Bench Press for Triceps (6 sets= 13 reps, 13, 11, 11, 11, 15)
1st week weight:
2nd week weight:
3rd week weight:
4th week weight:

F. Lat Pulldown (6 sets= 13 reps, 13, 11, 11, 11, 15)
1st week weight:
2nd week weight:
3rd week weight:
4th week weight:

G. Bicep Curl (6 sets= 13 reps, 13, 11, 11, 11, 15)
1st week weight:
2nd week weight:
3rd week weight:
4th week weight:

H. Cardio (Stationary Bike or Moderate Pace Jog)
10-15 minutes

End of Exercise

PHASE II.
Date:
Duration: 2 hours or less
Current weight in Kg.:
End- Goal: *Lean Body Mass*
CHEST and TRICEPS
First Day and Fourth Day
A. Warm –Up (Light Stretching) 3 minutes

B. Flat Barbell Press (6 sets= 13 reps, 13, 11, 11, 11, 15)
1st week weight:
2nd week weight:
3rd week weight:
4th week weight:

C. Incline Barbell Press (6 sets= 13 reps, 13, 11, 11, 11, 15)
1st week weight:
2nd week weight:
3rd week weight:
4th week weight:

D. Decline Barbell Press (6 sets= 13 reps, 13, 11, 11, 11, 15)
1st week weight:
2nd week weight:
3rd week weight:
4th week weight:

E. Flat Dumbell Flyes (6 sets= 13 reps, 13, 11, 11, 11, 15)
1st week weight:
2nd week weight:
3rd week weight:
4th week weight:

F. Close-Grip Barbell Press (6 sets= 13 reps, 13, 11, 11, 11, 15)
1st week weight:
2nd week weight:
3rd week weight:
4th week weight:

G. Cable Pulldown (6 sets= 13 reps, 13, 11, 11, 11, 15)
1st week weight:
2nd week weight:
3rd week weight:

4th week weight:

H. Tricep Extension (6 sets= 13 reps, 13, 11, 11, 11, 15)
1st week weight:
2nd week weight:
3rd week weight:
4th week weight:

I. Rope Pulldown (6 sets= 13 reps, 13, 11, 11, 11, 15)
1st week weight:
2nd week weight:
3rd week weight:
4th week weight:

J. Cardio (Stationary Bike or Moderate Pace Jog)
10-15 minutes
End of Exercise

PHASE II.
Date:
Duration: 2 hours or less
Current weight in Kg.:
End- Goal: *Lean Body Mass*
BACK and BICEPS
Second Day and Fifth Day
A. Warm –Up (Light Stretching) 3 minutes

B. Barbell Row (6 sets= 13 reps, 13, 11, 11, 11, 15)
1st week weight:
2nd week weight:
3rd week weight:
4th week weight:

C. T-bar Row (6 sets= 13 reps, 13, 11, 11, 11, 15)
1st week weight:
2nd week weight:
3rd week weight:
4th week weight:

D. Dumbbell Row (6 sets= 13 reps, 13, 11, 11, 11, 15)
1st week weight:
2nd week weight:
3rd week weight:
4th week weight:

E. Lat pull-down (6 sets= 13 reps, 13, 11, 11, 11, 15)
1st week weight:
2nd week weight:
3rd week weight:
4th week weight:

F. Seated machine Row (6 sets= 13 reps, 13, 11, 11, 11, 15)
1st week weight:
2nd week weight:
3rd week weight:
4th week weight:

G. Inclined Bicep curl (6 sets= 13 reps, 13, 11, 11, 11, 15)
1st week weight:
2nd week weight:
3rd week weight:
4th week weight:

H. Barbell curl (6 sets= 13 reps, 13, 11, 11, 11, 15)
1st week weight:
2nd week weight:
3rd week weight:
4th week weight:

I. machine bicep curl (6 sets= 13 reps, 13, 11, 11, 11, 15)
1st week weight:
2nd week weight:
3rd week weight:
4th week weight:

J. Cardio (Stationary Bike or Moderate Pace Jog)
10-15 minutes

End of Exercise

PHASE II.
Date:
Duration: 2 hours or less
Current weight in Kg.:
End- Goal: *Lean Body Mass*
SHOULDER and LEGS
Third Day and Sixth Day
A. Warm –Up (Light Stretching) 3 minutes

B. Squat (6 sets= 13 reps, 13, 11, 11, 11, 15)
1st week weight:
2nd week weight:
3rd week weight:
4th week weight:

C. Leg Press (6 sets= 13 reps, 13, 11, 11, 11, 15)
1st week weight:
2nd week weight:
3rd week weight:
4th week weight:

D. Leg curl (6 sets= 13 reps, 13, 11, 11, 11, 15)
1st week weight:
2nd week weight:
3rd week weight:
4th week weight:

E. Calf Raise (6 sets= 13 reps, 13, 11, 11, 11, 15)
1st week weight:
2nd week weight:
3rd week weight:
4th week weight:

F. Barbell military press (6 sets= 13 reps, 13, 11, 11, 11, 15)
1st week weight:
2nd week weight:
3rd week weight:
4th week weight:

G. Dumbell press (6 sets= 13 reps, 13, 11, 11, 11, 15)
1st week weight:
2nd week weight:
3rd week weight:
4th week weight:

H. Side lateral raise (6 sets= 13 reps, 13, 11, 11, 11, 15)
1st week weight:
2nd week weight:
3rd week weight:
4th week weight:

I. Back lateral raise (6 sets= 13 reps, 13, 11, 11, 11, 15)
1st week weight:
2nd week weight:
3rd week weight:

4th week weight:

J. Barbell Shrug (6 sets= 13 reps, 13, 11, 11, 11, 15)
1st week weight:
2nd week weight:
3rd week weight:
4th week weight:
K. Cardio (Stationary Bike or Moderate Pace Jog)
10-15 minutes

End of Exercise

PHASE III.
Date:
Duration: 2 hours or less
Current weight in Kg.:
End- Goal: ***Lean Body Mass***
CHEST and TRICEPS
First Day and Fourth Day
A. Warm –Up (Light Stretching) 3 minutes

B. Flat Barbell Press (5 sets= 11 reps, 11, 9, 9, 13)
1st week weight:
2nd week weight:
3rd week weight:
4th week weight:

C. Incline Barbell Press (5 sets= 11 reps, 11, 9, 9, 13)
1st week weight:
2nd week weight:
3rd week weight:
4th week weight:

D. Decline Barbell Press (5 sets= 11 reps, 11, 9, 9, 13)
1st week weight:
2nd week weight:
3rd week weight:
4th week weight:

E. Flat Dumbell Flyes   (5 sets= 11 reps, 11, 9, 9, 13)
1st week weight:
2nd week weight:
3rd week weight:
4th week weight:

F. Close-Grip Barbell Press (5 sets= 11 reps, 11, 9, 9, 13)

1st week weight:
2nd week weight:
3rd week weight:
4th week weight:

G. Cable Pulldown (5 sets= 11 reps, 11, 9, 9, 13)
1st week weight:
2nd week weight:
3rd week weight:
4th week weight:

H. Tricep Extension (5 sets= 11 reps, 11, 9, 9, 13)
1st week weight:
2nd week weight:
3rd week weight:
4th week weight:

I.Rope Pulldown (5 sets= 11 reps, 11, 9, 9, 13)
1st week weight:
2nd week weight:
3rd week weight:
4th week weight:

J. Cardio (Stationary Bike or Moderate Pace Jog)
10-15 minutes

End of Exercise

PHASE III.
Date:
Duration: 2 hours or less
Current weight in Kg.:
End- Goal: *Lean Body Mass*
BACK and BICEPS
Second Day and Fifth Day
A. Warm –Up (Light Stretching) 3 minutes

B. Barbell Row (5 sets= 11 reps, 11, 9, 9, 13)
1st week weight:
2nd week weight:
3rd week weight:
4th week weight:

C. T-bar Row (5 sets= 11 reps, 11, 9, 9, 13)
1st week weight:
2nd week weight:
3rd week weight:
4th week weight:

D. Dumbbell Row (5 sets= 11 reps, 11, 9, 9, 13)
1st week weight:
2nd week weight:
3rd week weight:
4th week weight:

E. Lat pull-down (5 sets= 11 reps, 11, 9, 9, 13)
1st week weight:
2nd week weight:
3rd week weight:
4th week weight:

F. Seated machine Row (5 sets= 11 reps, 11, 9, 9, 13)
1st week weight:
2nd week weight:
3rd week weight:
4th week weight:

G. Inclined Bicep curl (5 sets= 11 reps, 11, 9, 9, 13)
1st week weight:
2nd week weight:
3rd week weight:
4th week weight:

H. Barbell curl (5 sets= 11 reps, 11, 9, 9, 13)
1st week weight:
2nd week weight:
3rd week weight:
4th week weight:

I. machine bicep curl (5 sets= 11 reps, 11, 9, 9, 13)
1st week weight:
2nd week weight:
3rd week weight:
4th week weight:

J. Cardio (Stationary Bike or Moderate Pace Jog)
10-15 minutes
End of Exercise

PHASE III.
Date:
Duration: 2 hours or less
Current weight in Kg.:
End- Goal: ***Lean Body Mass***
SHOULDER and LEGS
Third Day and Sixth Day
A. Warm –Up (Light Stretching) 3 minutes

B. Squat (5 sets= 11 reps, 11, 9, 9, 13)
1st week weight:
2nd week weight:
3rd week weight:
4th week weight:

C. Leg Press (5 sets= 11 reps, 11, 9, 9, 13)
1st week weight:
2nd week weight:
3rd week weight:
4th week weight:

D. Leg curl (5 sets= 11 reps, 11, 9, 9, 13)
 1st week weight:
2nd week weight:
3rd week weight:
4th week weight:

E. Calf Raise (5 sets= 11 reps, 11, 9, 9, 13)
1st week weight:
2nd week weight:
3rd week weight:
4th week weight:

F. Barbell military press (5 sets= 11 reps, 11, 9, 9, 13)
1st week weight:
2nd week weight:
3rd week weight:
4th week weight:

G. Dumbell press (5 sets= 11 reps, 11, 9, 9, 13)
1st week weight:
2nd week weight:
3rd week weight:
4th week weight:

H. Side lateral raise (5 sets= 11 reps, 11, 9, 9, 13)
1st week weight:
2nd week weight:
3rd week weight:
4th week weight:

I. Back lateral raise (5 sets= 11 reps, 11, 9, 9, 13)
1st week weight:
2nd week weight:
3rd week weight:
4th week weight:

J. Barbell Shrug (5 sets= 11 reps, 11, 9, 9, 13)
1st week weight:
2nd week weight:
3rd week weight:
4th week weight:
K. Cardio (Stationary Bike or Moderate Pace Jog)
10-15 minutes

End of Exercise

PHASE IV.
Date:
Duration: 2 hours or less
Current weight in Kg.:
End- Goal: ***Lean Body Mass***
CHEST and TRICEPS
First Day and Fourth Day
A. Warm –Up (Light Stretching) 3 minutes

B. Flat Barbell Press (6 sets= 13 reps, 13, 11, 11, 11, 15)
1st week weight:
2nd week weight:
3rd week weight:
4th week weight:

C. Incline Barbell Press (6 sets= 13 reps, 13, 11, 11, 11, 15)
1st week weight:
2nd week weight:
3rd week weight:
4th week weight:

D. Decline Barbell Press (6 sets= 13 reps, 13, 11, 11, 11, 15)
1st week weight:
2nd week weight:

3rd week weight:
4th week weight:

E. Flat Dumbell Flyes (6 sets= 13 reps, 13, 11, 11, 11, 15)
1st week weight:
2nd week weight:
3rd week weight:
4th week weight:

F. Close-Grip Barbell Press (6 sets= 13 reps, 13, 11, 11, 11, 15)
1st week weight:
2nd week weight:
3rd week weight:
4th week weight:

G. Cable Pulldown (6 sets= 13 reps, 13, 11, 11, 11, 15)
1st week weight:
2nd week weight:
3rd week weight:
4th week weight:

H. Tricep Extension (6 sets= 13 reps, 13, 11, 11, 11, 15)
1st week weight:
2nd week weight:
3rd week weight:
4th week weight:

I. Rope Pulldown (6 sets= 13 reps, 13, 11, 11, 11, 15)
1st week weight:
2nd week weight:
3rd week weight:
4th week weight:

J. Cardio (Stationary Bike or Moderate Pace Jog)
10-15 minutes

End of Exercise

PHASE IV.
Date:
Duration: 2 hours or less
Current weight in Kg.:
End- Goal: *Lean Body Mass*
BACK and BICEPS
Second Day and Fifth Day
A. Warm –Up (Light Stretching) 3 minutes

B. Barbell Row (6 sets= 13 reps, 13, 11, 11, 11, 15)
1st week weight:
2nd week weight:
3rd week weight:
4th week weight:

C. T-bar Row (6 sets= 13 reps, 13, 11, 11, 11, 15)
1st week weight:
2nd week weight:
3rd week weight:
4th week weight:

D. Dumbbell Row (6 sets= 13 reps, 13, 11, 11, 11, 15)
1st week weight:
2nd week weight:
3rd week weight:
4th week weight:

E. Lat pull-down (6 sets= 13 reps, 13, 11, 11, 11, 15)
1st week weight:
2nd week weight:
3rd week weight:
4th week weight:

F. Seated machine Row (6 sets= 13 reps, 13, 11, 11, 11, 15)
1st week weight:
2nd week weight:
3rd week weight:
4th week weight:

G. Inclined Bicep curl (6 sets= 13 reps, 13, 11, 11, 11, 15)
1st week weight:
2nd week weight:
3rd week weight:
4th week weight:

H. Barbell curl (6 sets= 13 reps, 13, 11, 11, 11, 15)

1st week weight:
2nd week weight:
3rd week weight:
4th week weight:

I. machine bicep curl (6 sets= 13 reps, 13, 11, 11, 11, 15)
1st week weight:
2nd week weight:
3rd week weight:
4th week weight:

J. Cardio (Stationary Bike or Moderate Pace Jog)
10-15 minutes

End of Exercise

PHASE IV.
Date:
Duration: 2 hours or less
Current weight in Kg.:
End- Goal: *Lean Body Mass*
SHOULDER and LEGS
Third Day and Sixth Day
A. Warm –Up (Light Stretching) 3 minutes

B. Squat (6 sets= 13 reps, 13, 11, 11, 11, 15)
1st week weight:
2nd week weight:
3rd week weight:
4th week weight:

C. Leg Press (6 sets= 13 reps, 13, 11, 11, 11, 15)
1st week weight:
2nd week weight:
3rd week weight:
4th week weight:

D. Leg curl (6 sets= 13 reps, 13, 11, 11, 11, 15)
1st week weight:
2nd week weight:
3rd week weight:
4th week weight:

E. Calf Raise (6 sets= 13 reps, 13, 11, 11, 11, 15)
1st week weight:
2nd week weight:
3rd week weight:
4th week weight:

F. Barbell military press (6 sets= 13 reps, 13, 11, 11, 11, 15)
1st week weight:
2nd week weight:
3rd week weight:
4th week weight:

G. Dumbell press (6 sets= 13 reps, 13, 11, 11, 11, 15)
1st week weight:
2nd week weight:
3rd week weight:
4th week weight:

H. Machine Side lateral raise (6 sets= 13 reps, 13, 11, 11, 11, 15)
1st week weight:
2nd week weight:
3rd week weight:
4th week weight:

I. Machine Back lateral raise (6 sets= 13 reps, 13, 11, 11, 11, 15)
1st week weight:
2nd week weight:
3rd week weight:
4th week weight:

J. Barbell/Dumbell Shrug (6 sets= 13 reps, 13, 11, 11, 11, 15)
1st week weight:
2nd week weight:
3rd week weight:
4th week weight:
K. Cardio (Stationary Bike or Moderate Pace Jog)
10-15 minutes

End of Exercise

PHASE I.A
Date:
Duration: 2 hours or less
Current weight in Kg.:
End- Goal: ***Lean Body Mass***
A. Warm –Up (Light Stretching) 3 minutes

B. Squat (5 sets= 11 reps, 11, 9, 9, 13)
1st week weight:
2nd week weight:
3rd week weight:
4th week weight:

C. Military Press (5 sets= 11 reps, 11, 9, 9, 13)
1st week weight:
2nd week weight:
3rd week weight:
4th week weight:

D. Flat Bench Press (5 sets= 11 reps, 11, 9, 9, 13)
1st week weight:
2nd week weight:
3rd week weight:
4th week weight:

E. Close Grip Bench Press for Triceps (5 sets= 11 reps, 11, 9, 9, 13)
1st week weight:
2nd week weight:
3rd week weight:
4th week weight:

F. Lat Pulldown (5 sets= 11 reps, 11, 9, 9, 13)
1st week weight:
2nd week weight:
3rd week weight:
4th week weight:

G. Bicep Curl (5 sets= 11 reps, 11, 9, 9, 13)
1st week weight:
2nd week weight:
3rd week weight:
4th week weight:

H. Cardio (Stationary Bike or Moderate Pace Jog)
10-15 minutes
End of Exercise

Summary

Holistic approach in beginning an exercise program can be taxing. Finding the right guide that will provide essential information is important. There are six major body parts involve in a total development program. These are the Chest and Triceps, Back and Biceps, Shoulder and Legs.

A comprehensive program is provided so as to help you reach your body weight goal. The program is divided in to four phases. Phase I involves exercises that will help prepare the muscle groups acclimatize to working out. Phase II is divided into three set of exercises for the chest and triceps, back and biceps, shoulder and legs. Phase III is the same set of exercises from Phase II but the difference is that it is mostly heavy weights for the said months. The last phase, Phase IV is similar to Phase II exercises. Phase I.A involved with 5 sets and this time involve with heavier weights than Phase I exercises. The goal of the program is to provide muscle confusion for all the six major muscle groups involve in this exercise regimen.

II. Holistic Nutrition

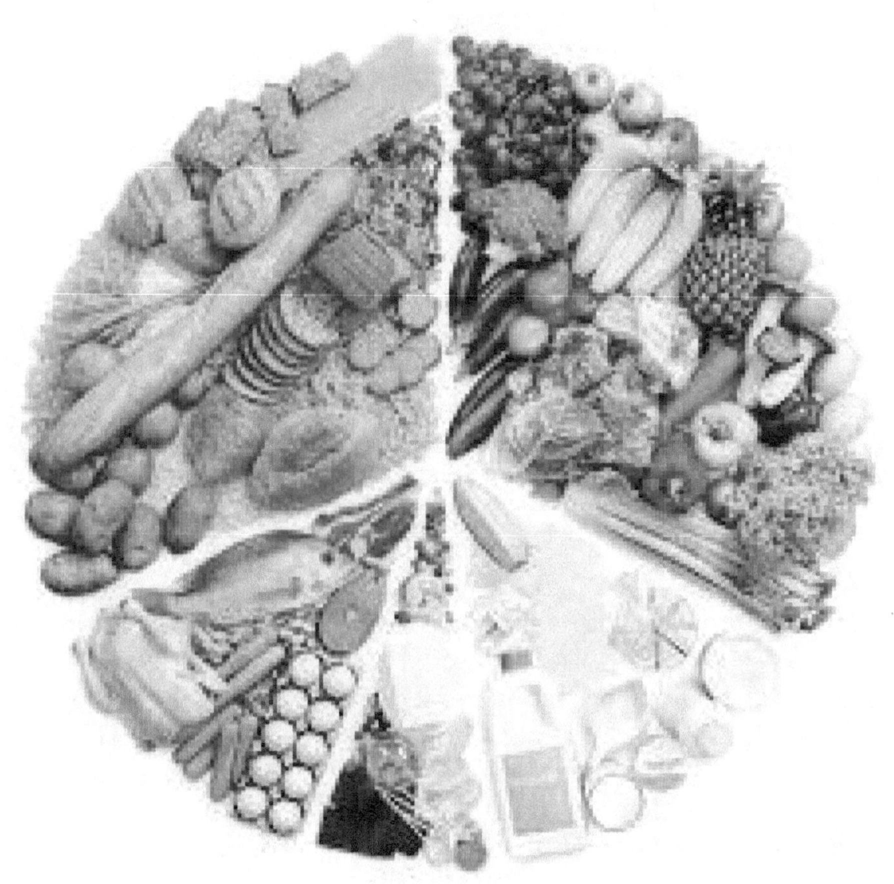

Chapter II. Holistic Nutrition

Importance of a Balanced Diet towards Achieving the Body you Desire

Seventy percent of your result in this manual is based on the food that you eat. For some people, this is the challenging part. It is important to note that food intake is the major factor in bringing out the body transformation you desire. Twenty percent is from your workout program and the other ten percent is in supplementation. This chapter will go in depth with the major food groups and sample balanced food plan that will help you reach your goal.

Major Food Groups

The major food groups are Proteins, Fats, and Carbohydrates. A lot of literature would suggest to increase protein intake so as to build muscle efficiently. But the downside of this is the high risk protein accumulation in the body resulting into kidney problems and increase uric acid. The main purpose of this plan is a BALANCE diet. Protein is important in building muscles. Carbohydrates as the main source of energy. Fats for alternative fuel source to keep the body in thermogenic condition.

Holistic Meal Plan

The sample meal plan presented here is for a one week period. You can add a variety to this plan so that it will not be boring on your part. The food items are a good source of good protein, complex carbohydrates, and healthy fats. Intermittent fasting (IF) can be applied on the fourth day and depends on your level of tolerance. Maximal time for fasting for this program is 4 to 6 hours maximum. Cheat meal for a day usually on the weekends but try to choose healthy food options and eat it all you can. Then resume on the usual food cycle for the entire week. Since I usually do my exercise program in the afternoon, I usually have my high carb 1.5 hours to 2 hours pre-workout.

Monday (First Day)

Cold water upon rising in the morning
Light jog for 10 to 15 mins.
Breakfast = 3 whole eggs + tuna + coffee
AM Snacks = 1 banana + whey protein
Lunch = Fish + Vegetables + rice
PM Snacks preworkout = any high carbs food + coffee
WORKOUT = whey protein + creatine /amino acid (depends on your budget)
 Post-workout = Gatorade or Chocolate Drink
Dinner = Chicken + rice + fruit of your choice

Beauty Rest = THE MOST IMPORTANT OF ALL LISTED ABOVE. It helps in muscle recovery and increase testosterone and growth hormones levels.

Tuesday (Second Day)

Cold water upon rising in the morning

Light jog for 10 to 15 mins.

Breakfast = 3 whole eggs + oats + coffee

AM Snacks = 1 fruit of choice + yogurt (it helps in good digestion)

Lunch = Chicken + Vegetables + rice

PM Snacks preworkout = any high carbs food + coffee

WORKOUT = whey protein + creatine /amino acid (depends on your budget)

 Post-workout = Gatorade or Chocolate Drink

Dinner = Fish +Vegetable dish + rice + fruit of your choice

Beauty Rest

Wednesday (Third Day)

Cold water upon rising in the morning

Light jog for 10 to 15 mins.

Breakfast = 3 whole eggs + chicken + coffee

AM Snacks = 1 banana + whey protein

Lunch = Fish + Vegetables + rice

PM Snacks preworkout = any high carbs food + coffee

WORKOUT = whey protein + creatine /amino acid (depends on your budget)

 Post-workout = Gatorade or Chocolate Drink

Dinner = Chicken + rice + fruit of your choice

Beauty Rest

Thursday (Intermittent Fasting) Fourth Day

Cold water upon rising in the morning

8 AM : Breakfast = coffee (fast until 12 PM)

12 PM : Lunch = Complex Carbs + Good Proteins + Dessert (any of your preference)

3 PM: Preworkout = 2 amino acid or 2 bcaa

Workout

Dinner = light dinner like oats with fruit.

Beauty rest

Friday (Fifth Day)

Cold water upon rising in the morning

Light jog for 10 to 15 mins.

Breakfast = 3 whole eggs + chicken + coffee

AM Snacks = pancake + whey protein

Lunch = Meat + Vegetables + rice

PM Snacks preworkout = any high carbs food + coffee

WORKOUT = whey protein + creatine /amino acid (depends on your budget)

Post-workout = Gatorade or Chocolate Drink

Dinner = Chicken + rice + fruit of your choice

Beauty Rest

Saturday (Sixth Day)

Cold water upon rising in the morning

Light jog for 10 to 15 mins.

Breakfast = 3 whole eggs + oats + coffee

AM Snacks = 1 fruit of choice + yogurt (it helps in good digestion)

Lunch = Chicken + Vegetables + rice

PM Snacks preworkout = any high carbs food + coffee

WORKOUT = whey protein + creatine /amino acid (depends on your budget)

 Post-workout = Gatorade or Chocolate Drink

Dinner = Fish +Vegetable dish + rice + fruit of your choice

Beauty Rest

Sunday (Seventh Day)

Rest Day

Eat all you Want/Can Day

Summary

This chapter deals with the holistic nutrition approach. It incorporates a balanced diet including protein, fats, and carbohydrates. It includes intermittent fasting approach and a eat all you can day which is more realistic than the meal plan available in literatures and in the market today. It gives you the option but in a very relaxed and non-intimidating way. It helps me keep my cravings in check and help me attain realistic outcomes rather that restricting myself and failing most of the time. With this meal plan, I was able to gain muscle or get lean depending on my current goal. Consult your physician before trying to incorporate intermittent fasting if you suspect you have any endocrine or hormone problems since it will alleviate some of its symptoms especially for the undiagnosed individuals. For the fit individuals, go ahead and try to journal your insights on your day to day progress.

III. Fundamentals of Supplementation

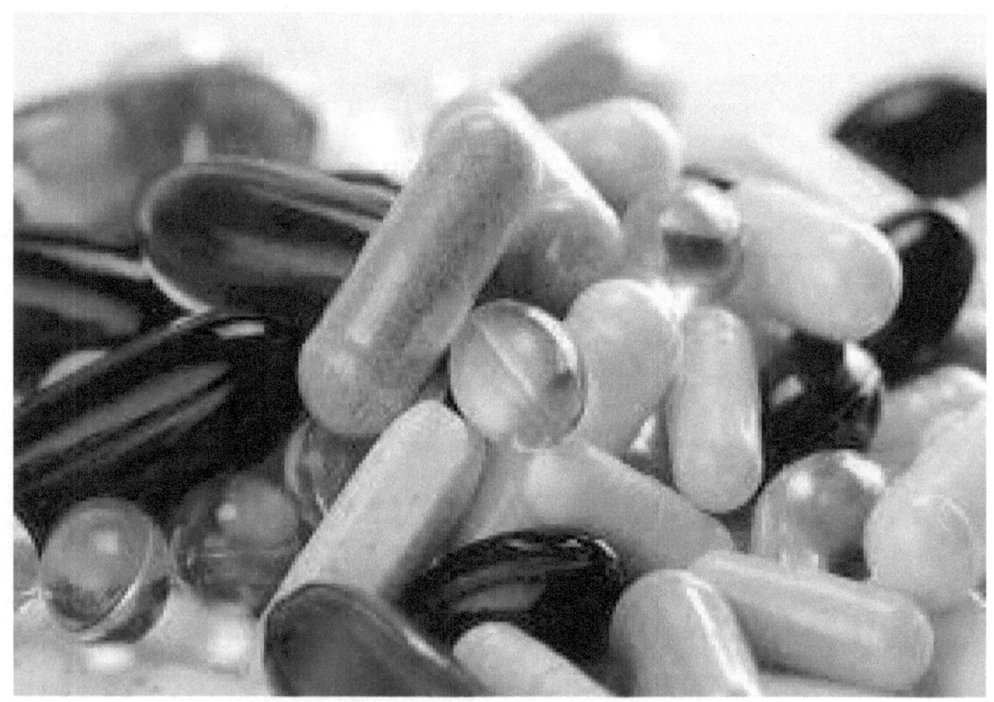

Chapter III. Fundamentals of Supplementation

Importance of Supplementation towards Visible Success

Supplementation is one of the underrated major contributors in the achievement of the body you aimed for. Different people have different views regarding the use of these products. Some will say that it is dangerous in a way that it will ruin your liver, kidneys, and may cause major health problems in the future. This is the reason why I wrote this book to provide you with firsthand experience in the use of these different supplements in the market. You don't need to suffer the consequences along the way. I will teach you the best supplements in the market and how to use it effectively and efficiently.

The second part of this chapter is dedicated to the use of testosterone supplements and growth hormones and my personal journey of using this product. And try to answer the questions, Do I really need it or do I stick with the old school supplementation? These questions will be answered as we go thru this manual. I am not recommending you to do the same but let your intelligence take its own course. Trust and listen to your body. As the old adage state, Experience is the Best Teacher.

Most Commonly Used Supplements in the Market

Different Supplements are already available in the market today. And sometimes it becomes tiring what products to choose from and what are the best supplements to take. Supplements are categorized either us a preworkout, Mid-workout, and Post-workout. Each supplements have different rationale why the best way to take it is preworkout, mid-workout, or post workout. Let us start with our preworkout supplements.

Preworkout supplements are taken before workout commence. Its main purpose is to give you energy and facilitate maximal muscular effort during the workout program. Most common preworkout products are Jack 3d, C4, and NOX. But based on my experience I stick to using BCAA usually 2 caps or 2tabs preworkout and a whey protein+creatine (depending on my budget) before working out. I find my muscle not that sore and I recover fast after an intense program.

Midworkout is taken during the workout program. This is important to provide your muscle with glucose to avoid muscle tearing and helps in providing a constant energy for the entire program. Commonly used midworkout supplement are glutamine but I stick with my whey protein+creatine combination.

Post workout supplement is important because it helps provide you with glucose to stabilize your blood sugar after a workout. Gatorade for electrolyte replacement is good. For me, a chocolate drink is the way to go. It's complete with nutrients and minerals for faster recovery.

Performance Enhancing Supplements (PES) Guide

I know you are excited for this part because this is the part that most of the people in gym will not admit about. The use of performance enhancing supplements is one of the most talked about forum in the internet. Different people have different insights on this matter. I tried the best in the market and YES the result is visible. That is the reason why people try to discourage you from using it because of its effect. But always remember, Great Power comes Great responsibility. After 8 years of working out, I hit Plateau and I did not make progress anymore and that's the reason why I tried personally this PES. I recorded my experiences and my observable changes for the entire 6 months cycle and I was able to conclude that it is EFFECTIVE. But the RESULTS is greater than the RISKS. After the cycle I did Post Cycle Therapy (PCT) to have my normal testosterone level production back. My Blood pressure is high and I am quiet irritable during the entire 6 months. But if you want to experience yourself, I will provide you with the detailed process on how to cycle safely and effectively.

Compendium of Balanced Supplementation

In this Testosterone Cycle I used T.Enanhate for the entire 6 months cycle. I used a 3 ml syringe. Each 10 ml vial is 250 mg/ml. You have to inject intramuscularly and better find a medical professional to assist you to avoid hematoma or untoward reaction. Injection is done 1 hour before workout.

First to Second week of the first month, start with 150 mg of T. enanhate three times per week. My schedule is every Tuesday, Thursday, and Friday. With 0.5 ml of T. Enanhate.

Third and Fourth week of the first month, increase T. enanhate to 250 mg per week. Schedule is the same as above. Avoid site infection all the time.

One month is equal to one cycle. Repeat process for the second cycle and end with the Third month of the third cycle and OFF.

After the third month, it's your choice to continue the cycle or discontinue.

Post Cycle Therapy (PCT)

This is done if you decide to discontinue the Testosterone cycle. The main purpose of this therapy is to resume your normal testosterone production because during the entire testosterone cycle, your body stopped producing normal testosterone because there is an abundant supply of it during the cycle. It is important to undergo PCT to avoid unwanted negative effects of testosterone cycle such as gynecomastia, shrinking of testicles, etc.

For my PCT program, I used Growth Hormone and Clomid for the entire month post testosterone cycle.

For the First and Second Week PCT, I have 0.05 cc of GH SQ + 1 tab Clomid.

During the Third and Fourth week, only Clomid 1 tab until the end of the month of the Post Cycle Therapy.

Summary

Supplementation is one of the underrated major contributors in the achievement of the body you aimed for. Different people have different views regarding the use of these products. Some will say that it is dangerous in a way that it will ruin your liver, kidneys, and may cause major health problems in the future. This is the reason why I wrote this book to provide you with firsthand experience in the use of these different supplements in the market. You don't need to suffer the consequences along the way. I will teach you the best supplements in the market and how to use it effectively and efficiently.

Different Supplements are already available in the market today. And sometimes it becomes tiring what products to choose from and what are the best supplements to take. Supplements are categorized either us a preworkout, Mid-workout, and Post-workout. Each supplements have different rationale why the best way to take it is preworkout, mid-workout, or post workout.

The use of performance enhancing supplements is one of the most talked about forum in the internet. Different people have different insights on this matter. I tried the best in the market and YES the result is visible. That is the reason why people try to discourage you from using it because of its effect. But always remember, Great Power comes with Great responsibility.